I0425936

The Professional Pilates Teacher's Handbook

Laurette Ryan
2013

Introduction and background....

The inspiration for writing this book has come to me through many years of mentoring and supporting new teachers. I have always tried to impart good self-care and business strategies to those teachers throughout the years whom I have had the blessing to assist. Much of what I have passed on has come from 30 plus years of experience in teaching movement as a career.

 I specifically got down to the task of writing this book after two pivotal events.

There are times in your life of large and small crossroads.

You travel along sometimes not even noticing you've passed through the crossroad and go right along never knowing a different journey was waiting down that intersection. There are times in your life when even the straightest smoothest road seems a burden to travel, that's when you should be ready for the crossroad!

So in my story I'm traveling down the smooth road. My business is busy, I'm doing what I love. (I'm really blessed to say that for over 30 years-I get up daily to a job I adore!) I happened to be at a Pilates conference having the time of my life with the people I love.... and then it happened !

Someone put to me a question, so profound .
It was like a quick hard slap in the face!
The kind of a question that to me, was like the alarm
clock of life -saying
WAKE UP. ! You might be living the life you dreamed
about living...
but time to stop and create a new more meaningful
dream.

So that person receives my deepest gratitude .

The question: **"What do you WANT to do? "**

It's a brilliant question and if I may.....let me ask
you that question too.

If you take some time and thoughtfully answer it, and
then go out and act on it...it will change and
possibly improve your life.

My answer: "Oh ,teach more workshops, grow my teacher
training program...."
I knew my answer was , well not the answer..

1.It was stuff I was already doing.

2.It held no challenge. The question made me see - I
had no direction - just drifting along on some good
currents.

Drifting is okay, for a little while but can get
monotonous, even when the sky is bright and the wind
is strong.

I was disturbed by my answer. It made me think.

I knew I wanted to continue to teach Pilates teachers - I love that. But above and beyond, I really had a desire to contribute something more. I wanted to give teachers something different, important and valuable. An insight that would improve their teaching and businesses.

Teaching teachers is something I do well, with my heart and soul. Exercises, theory, skills, my program does all that, but there was one thing more teachers came to me for …. advice.

Advice on fixing their bodies, fixing client relationship issues, building their businesses ,work environments and sometimes just to get fired-up again, to do their work.

The next pivotal event was what I started to notice around me.

 The conference I was at , was in a location less than desirable to people who prize their health.

I watched people who normally took great care of themselves starting to disintegrate, first physically, then emotionally.

It was really, quite predictable to me. The environment was energetically draining... seriously! draining **energy** from the body- in a real and noticeable sense.

Being sensitive to energy is part of who I am. So I saw this and I wondered, is there scientific information, data on this phenomena? Personally , I felt from experience, there are people ,places and events that sap your energy. Making someone's mood or energy level or even immunity drop low. BUT , had anyone set out to prove that.

So these 2 events took me to my current crossroad......

It is the place where I started to research, write about and teach teachers...how to be aware, mange their energy, deal with clients and create a business- THEY LOVE!

Preventing burnout starts with these steps in self-care.

Once you have defined your personal master-plan for teaching , one that keeps you smiling everyday, only then can you build a career, a business of your dreams.

So Part One of this book deals with setting parameters for self-care and Part Two is filled with tips and strategies to grow your business.

I hope you will be inspired and fired-up to live your dream life......

What do YOU want to do?
This may be your crossroads......

fondly- Laurette Ryan

Dedicated to all those who deem to ask profound questions.......

To: my dearest, Rebecca
With sincerest gratitude for an alert to a crossroads...

...also to a woman named, Laura, that I taught with, a thousand years ago, who once asked me another profound question, "Do you want to ride in the roller-coaster? Or would you rather drive it?"

and mostly dedicated to you-
the teacher, the one giving from your heart , soul and physical being. Trying your best , wanting to save everyone and sometimes losing yourself. You are so precious , so valuable -I wish you great rewards in this life and know that the greatest rewards are not the tangible ones, but instead the intangible, the whispers of the angels to your soul that say- Yes, you made the world better.....

Table of Contents:

Part One:

Part Two:

PART ONE:

The 4 Aspects of Self

You are a complex and beautifully
balanced human being.

Teaching movement, exercise and wellness to others
is noble, wonderful, exhausting, inspiring, fatiguing
and phenomenal.

In order to stay vibrant and successful in your
career you must take care of yourself. Keep your fire
burning and prevent burning out.

In your wonderful complexity consider this :you
teach- with your whole being.

Your whole being or whole self is comprised of at
least 4 distinct aspects.
The physical,rational/mental,emotional and energetic
"selves" or aspects.

PHYSICAL

MENTAL

EMOTIONAL

ENERGETIC

Taking care and consideration of these aspects is vital to your continued success.

Caring for your **Physical aspect** entails good daily self-care, body mechanics and a balanced healthy lifestyle.

Your **Rational/ mental aspect** includes direction for keeping the mind sharp and engaged in the teaching process.

Emotional aspects address issues of professional boundaries, logically navigating the professional relationship.

Finally the **Energetic aspect** of self deals with the science of the energetic body, the fascia, nervous system and energy, energy fields and frequencies and strategies to keep your energy clear and moving to balance yourself and your environment.

The Physical Aspect of Self

What is Body Mechanics?

Definition: Body mechanics studies muscular actions and the function of muscles in maintaining body posture. Knowledge from such studies is especially important in the prevention of injury during the performance of tasks that require the body to lift and move.

Good body mechanics as a movement teacher is essential. As we help others explore and improve their lifestyle body mechanics , we can unintentionally, put our own bodies at risk.

There are 3 aspects to good body mechanics for the movement teacher.

1. **Lifting and moving apparatus or equipment.**
2. **Assisting clients**
3. **Teaching posture**

Movement teachers generally consider themselves fit, sometimes very fit and often believe that the rules are for mere mortals.

They believe that they are so strong and invincible because of the work they do and embody, that they can cheat the rules, at least a little, and it will have no consequences for them.

They are mistaken!

Years of teaching have taught me, that not only is this an incorrect assumption, it is a dangerous one. Not only in the present moment where the offending motion/movement occurs, but years later after minor damage which seemingly healed or was only a nagging pain becomes the weak link in an aging body.

You see much to our chagrin, although your work will keep you moving and enjoying a life of physical fitness and pleasure longer than your peers, there are biological realities we all face.

As we age, and particularly after age forty, cell regeneration starts to slow. This means we heal and repair at a slower rate. Our bodies are constantly in a state of tearing down and building up. When you are young that building up phase is really in hyper-drive... but as you get older it levels off, and the re-building actually slows in relation to the tearing down. It's a fact- it's biology.

So you can accept this reality and work WITH the knowledge or ignore it and face the consequences. (By the way it doesn't matter how awesome and cool you are! It applies to EVERYONE)

Along with the knowledge that we are re-building at a slower rate and shouldn't do things that put us behind the curve intentionally, we need to understand that every old injury still may live within our fascial bed.

You may have been repairing and restoring quickly enough at age 25 or 35, not to notice the past injuries effects on the whole body but as you slow down, these weak links start to announce themselves.

This is good argument for not creating bad patterns at age 25... (this is the most challenging part of my message, because when you are 25 and feeling invincible - you can't imagine I'm speaking a truth here.

Not me! I won't allow myself to fall apart when I'm 40! I'm smarter and stronger- those people are just giving in!

I get it! I was YOU and let me re-iterate -it is not lack of willpower or drive that slows you down - it IS biology... science, fact!)

Be smart at 25 - you want your body to work well and with little discomfort till 95! Good maintenance is key!

So once you understand the biology, how do you create good strategies and movement rules for yourself that work?

Lifting and moving apparatus, equipment with good body mechanics seems like common sense.

 We have all heard the advice to bend the knees while lifting - this on the surface may alleviate some risk, but if we understand WHY bending the knees while lifting is a good idea, we can use this premise more effectively.

Most individuals as we know have tight hamstrings. If we bend forward and have tight hamstrings chances are the back will become very flexed.

This position of hanging forward dangling your body weight off the ligaments of the vertebral column - pushing discs posterior-ly is downright foolish to start with - when you couple that with adding a load-like lifting a weight or piece of equipment, you put the back in a very precarious position.

Additionally the load is generally positioned further from the center line of the body making the load in fact heavier...your center muscles will need to generate more force to move the load in order for you to remain upright.

So if you bend your knees while lifting - you are taking some of the strain off the back... the load you may be lifting will be in closer proximity to your center. But you can still be putting your spine in danger if you are flexing it forward and hanging off your vertebral joints.

Axial Elongation or Spinal Lift can appropriately engage the spinals before forward bending. The action of lifting, lengthening and activating your spine BEFORE flexing it, in order to distribute the workload evenly.

 Another strategy (and my preferred) is to keep the back straight while lifting . Bend the knees , keep the back long and straight and lift the object. The act of keep the back straight while lifting is strengthening and builds strong core as well.

Some instances of using this technique may be obvious. Lifting equipment, weights or even searching in a storage bin for a theraband or such.

Some instances may not be so obvious.

Such as :
Adjusting equipment.

   *For Pilates teachers this can mean adjusting the headrest or springs, or foot-strap or footbar.

 Getting handles and foot loops., springs from below

    *For other Movement teachers getting out mats, weights,cardio-steps, fixing benches and handles, moving equipment.

 *Bodyworkers carrying tables.

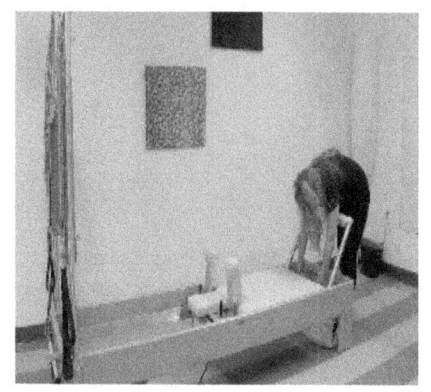 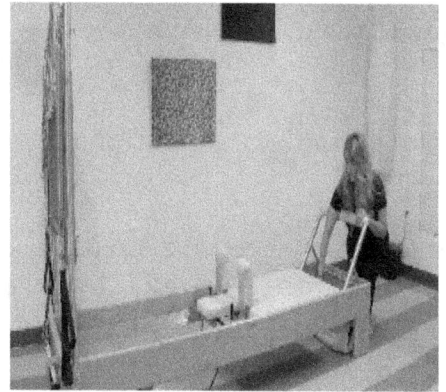

Don't !   Do!

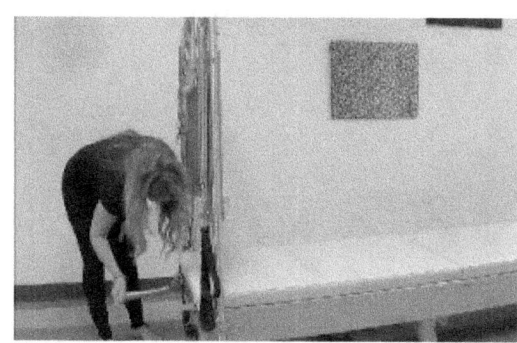

Don't !

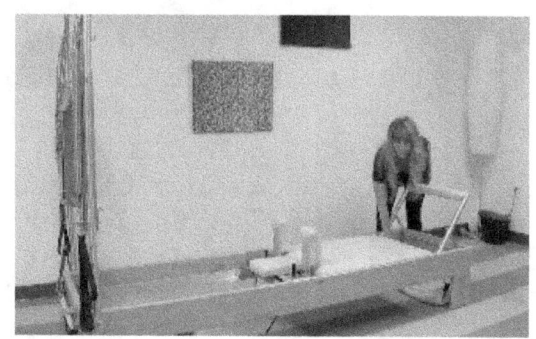

Do!

Assisting clients

There are many times we will be physically assisting clients.

Depending on the clients physical state merely getting on and off an apparatus, table or machine could require assistance.

At ALL times, our first priority must be client safety for liability reasons.

Properly explaining how you want the client to get from point A to point B is your first line of defense.

Then explain HOW you may be assisting them. ie: I will hold your hand and you will do XYZ.

Always explain what your physical assistance will be. Make sure they are comfortable with that. ..." Is that okay?, do you understand?"

For some clients your just reaching out and touching them could be so unexpected that they take you both down!

You must always keep a careful watch on the client and be anticipating their next move. Being distracted during a session is as dangerous for you as it is for the client.

Use the rules of good body mechanics when adjusting or assisting your client- flexing forward, hanging out on your spine or trying to lift or move them is a definite NO.

When assisting during a difficult exercise, you must stand with good form, weight even in both legs, back tall, shoulder girdle activated in the appropriate manner and MOST of all eyes open, attentively.

You **could** save your body by NOT assisting when a client is about to, or has taken a fall or cannot return their own bodies to a safe position but chances are you **will** jump in there and help...

If you are ready with the body prepared-<u>attentive,</u> you will be less likely to hurt yourself.

(not being attentive IS negligent and you can be liable)

Teaching posture

We know as teachers of movement that things we do
repetitively in our lives leave their imprint in our
bodies.

If we stand on one leg, hip jutting out, hands on
hips, ribcage shifted to the opposite side, we are
making a fairly unsustainable pattern of imbalance in
our muscles, tendons, ligaments, bones and fascia
that will eventually become discomfort and then pain.

If we do this long enough or bodies- muscles and yes
even bone will start to morph and change into this
unbalanced shape. Making it all the more difficult to
undo.

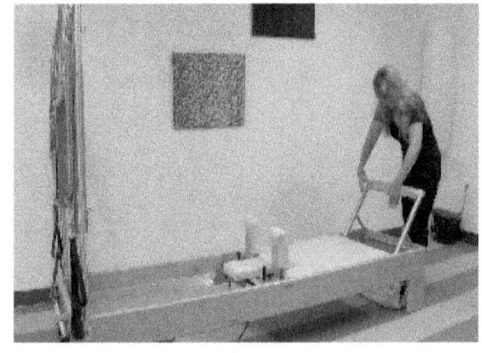

DON'T !

BETTER TEACHING POSTURES

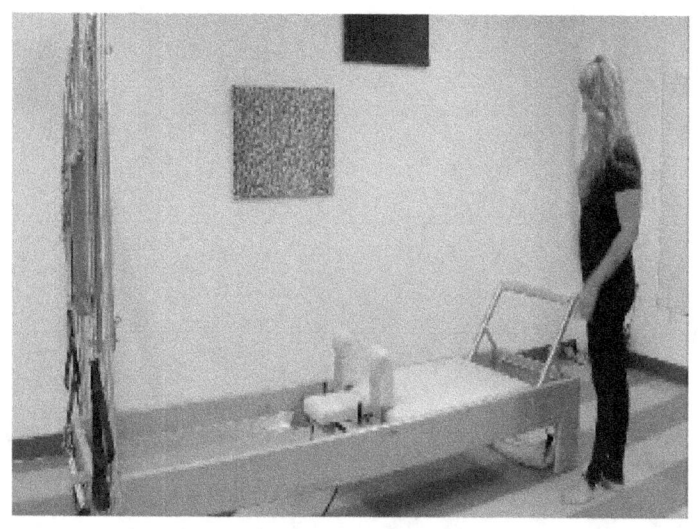

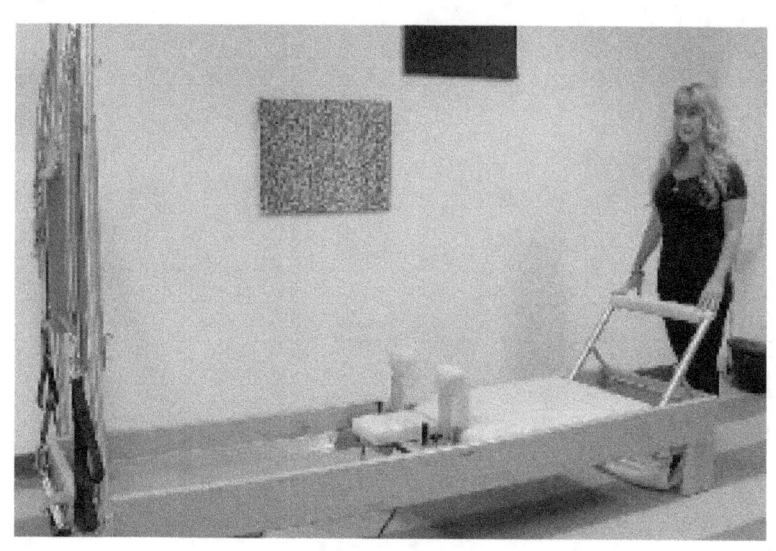

25

OVERALL POSTURAL HABITS

You know you're bad habits. Standing to one side or slouching or legs overly externally rotating or whatever it is. You may also realize that when you are tired or focused on something else (like someone else's body) you can easily fall back into these habits.

What are your bad posture habits?

Neck?

_____

Upper Back?

_____

Lower Back?

_____

Pelvis?

_____

Legs?

_____

Knees?

_____

Feet?

_____

Do you favor standing on one leg?

_____

Do you tip your head to one side?

_____

During a session of teaching we may allow these
ineffective posture strategies to creep in and we may
be holding our bodies in detrimental positions for
long periods of time. In fact, imprinting these
postures in our neuro-muscular memory.

Teach with good alignment in our own bodies helps the
student internalize on a visual level- good body
alignment. Think in terms of modeling an example you
would like to see them replicate.

This not only assists your student, the reason you do
it - is a selfish one- your saving your own body !

DEMONSTRATIVE TEACHING

Teaching mat, or calisthenics or dance has some other pitfalls. If you demonstrate while you teach, as in you perform the exercises, combinations with the student or students do you contort your own body to watch them as you do it?

Do you lie on a mat with your head turned sideways to watch while you do the exercise? Or do you model it exactly as you would have them do , with head and neck in perfect alignment, focused on your form and your form alone?

There are a couple of issues here:

1. If you are totally focused on performing the exercises/moves in your body- you are not attentive to your students...
2. You are attentive to your students and you ARE putting your body at risk....
3. Teachers are the best cheaters! You can make it look perfect - when you know on the inside you are absolutely NOT doing what you're asking the student to do- ohhh but it looks sooo good!

**If you teach for your own workout.... STOP and realize that is not truly teaching, it might be instructing (which has it's merits) but it's not teaching.... it's workout with me! I'm fun! Compete against me -motivation! It has it's place- but it's not really teaching.

So teachers- beware of demonstration teaching- if you must - Do this: you show with good form while they watch and then they do- and you watch.

ATTENTIVE TEACHING

The next area to examine is how you position you're body to attentively teach. Do you spend long hours stooping over a person on a piece of equipment. Looking down at their bodies, or maybe even looking sideways at their bodies.

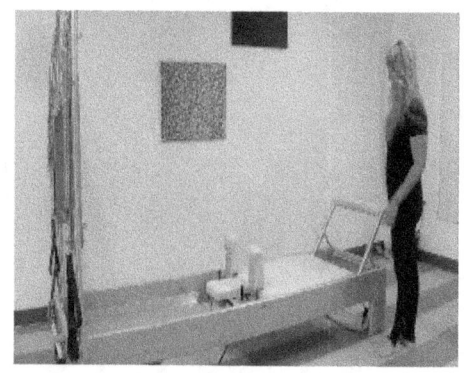
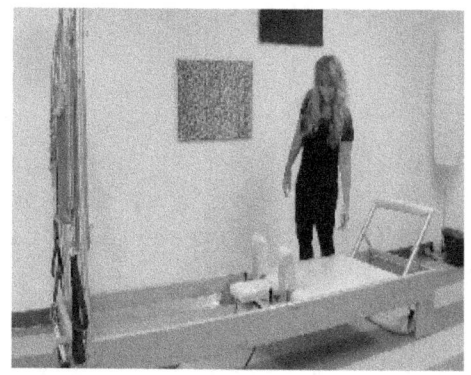

DO   DON'T

29

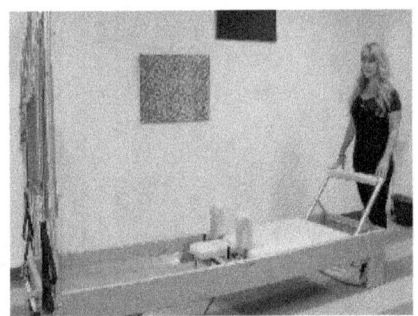

Do!

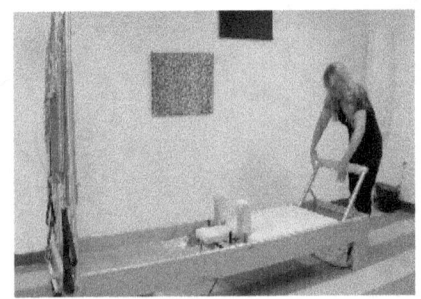

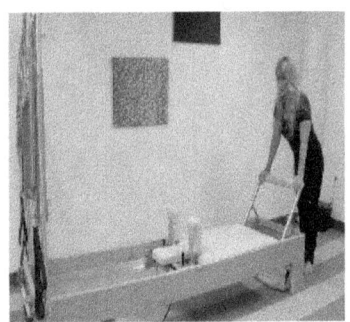

DON'T !   DO !

The good news is you are a teacher of good movement
and form - so you can undo whatever it is that you
might be doing while attentively teaching.

You just need to be aware of it and how much time you
are spending in these less than satisfactory body
positions.

Just like many jobs in today's society, we are
stooping forward from the head neck and shoulders .
Rounding the thoracic spine, shortening the chest
muscles, over stretching the upper back. It's not
just that poor office worker that we look at with
such pity - It could be YOU!

We know the prescription for this... thoracic
extension, strengthening and stretching and we should
take heed and make certain we get a good dose.

It is impossible and impractical to expect to be able
to teach and not look at your clients/students body
while the are lying down. However one aspect we maybe
able to ameliorate is the sideways glancing.

If you always stand to one side of your client …. be
sure to start standing on the other . This will feel
a bit uncomfortable at first - you may even feel
unable to see them properly. Seriously one eye does
focus better.

POSTURE RX for the TEACHER

The De-Slumper-

Stand against a wall. Heels and Shoulders touching
the wall. Put your hands below the navel -belt line,
pull the abdominals in and up. Touch the occiput (low
back of the head) to the wall (you might make a
horrible double chin) -hold for 10 seconds- repeat 3
times.

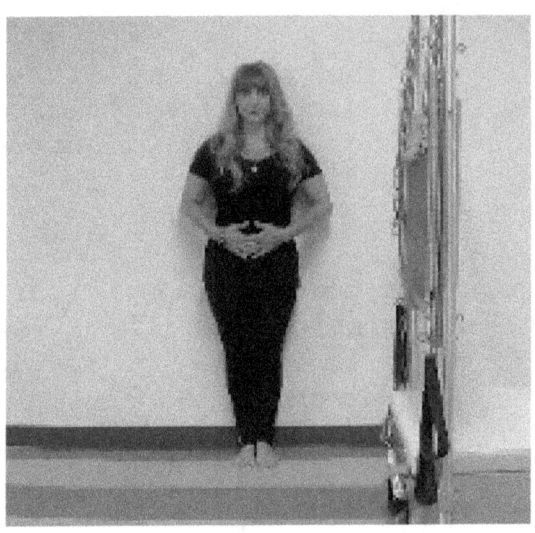

The Sway-

Standing -shift the weight side to side- hold on the right leg 1 to 2 minutes and then sway to the left 1-2 minutes...if one leg struggles a bit or seems more fatigued -notice this and work to strengthen that side.

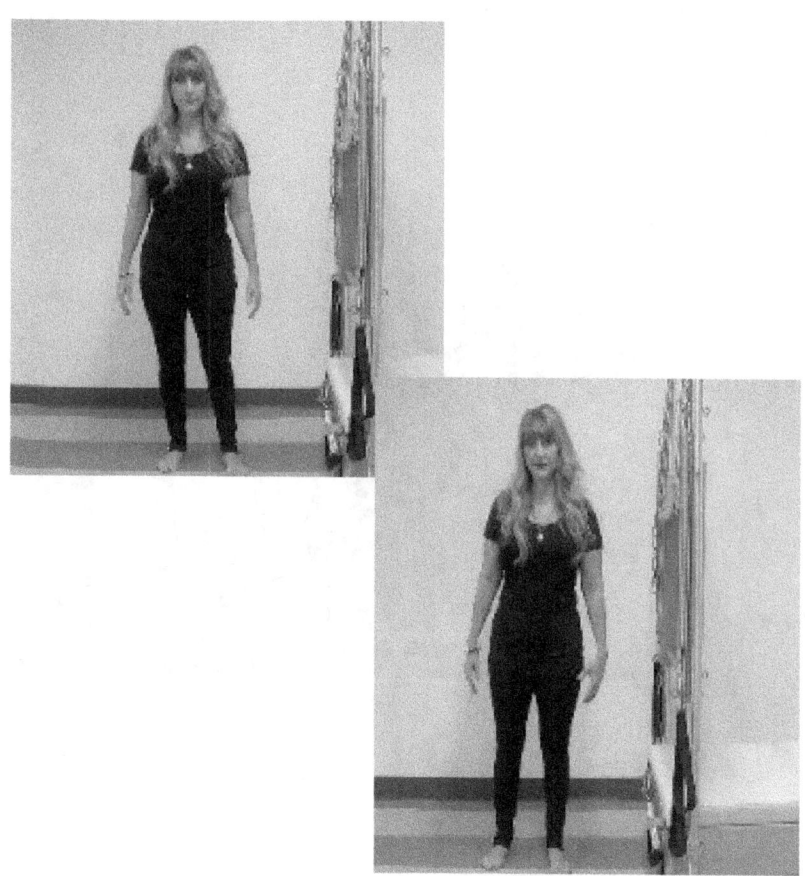

Ball Bounces-

Nourish the Spine- Sit on a stability ball a lightly bounce up and down softly and rhythmically. This encourages movement of fluids to hydrate the discs-keeping them healthy and happy!

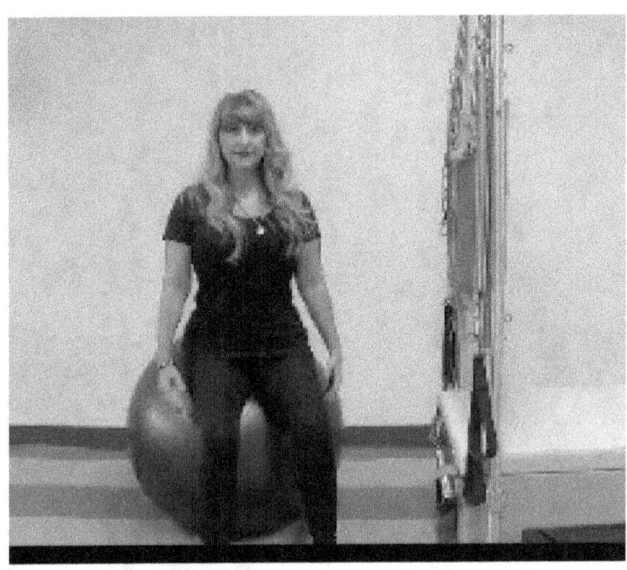

Self Care: Balanced Lifestyle!

Physical maintenance, self-care should be easy. For many teachers it involves merely taking your own advice!

Nutrition!

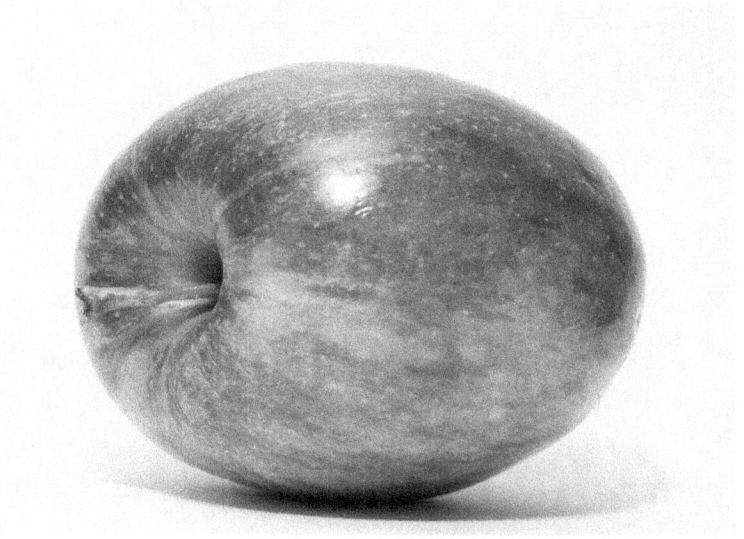

Do you tell students to eat well? Getting a proper amount of fruits and veggies, drinking water, proper amounts of protein, fats and carbs- Whatever your advice is...Do you actually follow it? It you preach it and believe what your saying is true - then you should!

Eating properly is essential to functioning properly!

If you are off track because of a busy hectic schedule- start tracking your food intake- treat yourself the way you expect your students to treat themselves, if they wish to be healthy.

Being unwilling to understand your bodies need for a nourishing diet will lead to fatigue, burn out and ill-health.

ZZZzzzzzzz's

Do you get enough rest?

Adults vary in the amount of sleep and rest they need. You need to explore what amount is correct for your system.

And maybe you are also a candidate for a siesta- a little afternoon power-nap!

If that is what makes you feel revived and energized to do your work , then you must make it part of your schedule.

Not receiving the proper amount of sleep can lead to:

weight gain

lethargy

heart disease

diabetes

headache

delayed reaction time

depression

to name a few....

Journal :

What type of diet is appropriate for me- I feel my
best when I eat like this............

The amount of sleep I need is.......

Rest is a Constructive activity. A smart teacher will insist on getting their sleep needs met. Sleep is necessary for our brains to work properly. It leads to impaired memory and physical performance. We are not able to carry out complex motor or learning tasks.

 Deep sleep coincides with the release of several hormones, such as growth hormone in children and young adults. Many of the body's cells also show increased growth and repair of damage from factors like stress and UV rays during deep sleep.Deep sleep seems to be particularly important for brain recovery during sleep and may be associated with improved performance and memory that results from sleep after learning.

Our bodies are our tools. You must rest and move your body in the most sensible way. That being said when is the last time you took a class or lesson , or did movement -just for you?

Having a good movement experience regularly for your body is inoperative. Movement can be and should be healing and restorative. You should leave any movement experience, workout or lesson feeling better than when you started- truly if that's not the case - you are doing something wrong. Getting the right amount and type of movement into your body is as important as the right amount and type of food and the right amount and type of rest.

Schedules are important. Set clear boundaries for when you teach, when you eat, when you rest and when you move-just for yourself -and stick to it. A regular schedule is the best way to guard against letting your good physical health management strategies fall off the tracks - or when they do - a schedule is a great way to get back on the track.

Balancing and managing your diet, rest, and movement/exercise is essential to caring for your physical body.... If you destroy your own physical health not only are your days numbered to teach, you really have no business teaching others to balance their physical health and fitness. Do you?

The Rational/Mental Aspect Self

Keeping the Mind Sharp Wards off Burn-out.

Continuing education in your field keeps you ahead of
the pack in terms of competition, but it also keeps
you mentally tuned-in and interested in what you are
doing.

Attending lectures, workshops or other teachers
classes keeps your perspective fresh. It will also
enhance your skills and give you new tools and tricks
to make your work more effective,challenging or
deepen the clients experience.

You should make a regular schedule of learning new
things monthly- by reading articles or books, viewing
videos,taking a class AND at least once per year
attend a major conference or workshop offering
-taking workshops with someone new. You may love your
mentors but expanding your horizons growing beyond
your supposed limits will give you a jolt of
inspiration and drive.

Playing increases brain power and creativity. It's a
fact- when is the last time you just played...not at
your work, but something completely different.. a new
sport, activity or just a romp somewhere. Play
increases hormones that reduces stress and decrease
hormones which are stress-related. Stress reduction
is associated with better function of the brain
during learning activities. Want to be smarter and
more relaxed- Go outside and play awhile!

When you are involved in repetitive activities -giving every client the same workout day after day - you actually become less focused, less attentive and your higher critical thinking skills fall into decline. Even if the movements are the same - find a new twist, nuance and perspective to keep yourself inspired and effectual.

Do you want to keep your self mentally sharp? Take the following steps:

Exercise:

This month learn one brand-new thing per week and list:

1._____

2._____

3._____

4._____

Give yourself permission to play everyday for one
week for at least 10 minutes (preferably longer but
if you haven't been playing- it's a start)
If you already have an activity or sport that is play
- try a new one!

What did you do?

Sunday through Saturday keep a list:
and jot your feelings.....if you haven't been playing
feeling guilty might be your response. Acknowledge
this and then allow yourself to take in the fact that
"play" restores your brain function and health and is
as necessary as food and water to every human being..

My "Playlist"!

Exercise:

Take one movement and find a completely new way to teach it. Practice it in your own body and note subtleties and nuance you sense in your own movement...

Work with another teacher and have them teach it to you or watch videos and read more about the anatomy involved....

See how many ways your new discoveries can be applied in other similar movements.

Mentally recharging is one key to maintaining your enthusiasm for teaching , if you lose your enthusiasm- you will soon be losing students too. If you're bored with you- how can they not be?

So far we have addressed the physical and mental aspects of you as a teacher - if you are not engaged in good self-care in these two areas, you are probably close to or completely burnt out already- address these aspects as best you are able and then you have a foundation to add the next two important aspects of self to.

The Emotional Aspect of Self

There are so many aspects to being a professional in any given field. Many of these are outlined in our teacher training manuals and at times you could say most of it is common sense... be discreet, be on time, dress appropriately.

Did you realize this is only the tip of what could be a very dangerous iceberg for your career? Did you know that if you understand all aspects of being a professional and having professional relationships with your students, you will be more successful, feel accomplished in your work and prevent burnout?

First off, we all need to realize that there are times our behavior could be better. All of us! We need to own it and resolve to get better at maintaining professional standards- for the benefit of not only our students, but also ourselves. When you have clients or students, maintaining professional boundaries and standards is crucial to your continued success and to managing your energy in order to prevent burn out. Adhering to a "professional" scope of practice, ethics and behaviors is not only good for your client welfare- but also compulsory for your welfare as well.

You must, in your practice create the "safe space" or "safe container" . That means that you are entering into a professional and therapeutic relationship with the client, and there are hard and fast rules that you must follow in order to have your client progress, improve and feel supported in the relationship.

Loose boundaries make the client unlikely to succeed and leave you burnt out.

Your rules and policies must be clear and understood, you should do no harm physically or emotionally and understand what types of situations pose a risk.

So many wellness "professionals" really have no idea that certain behaviors may be limiting their success . More and more I see teachers in my own profession of Pilates falling into these ethical pitfalls - it is also rampant in fields like massage therapy, personal training, yoga and more.

SELLING THINGS:

You must realize that if you are someone's Pilates teacher- chances are they already regard you as a professional of sorts- *(if they don't -you will know it by their inconsiderate behavior - late cancels, no shows, late payment- more on this shortly)*

But- if they regard you as "their" teacher you have entered a special type of relationship, a therapeutic relationship.

In this relationship -they trust your opinion, they think of you as the expert, they may not ever question your direction even if it's not in their best interest.

Sometimes you will recognize this by the way they start to ask you about medical conditions beyond the scope of your practice. So with this special type of relationship you are now obligated to consider that you may have a great deal of influence over them.

It is your responsibility and I feel, a sacred obligation, to be sure that you do not haphazardly use your undue influence over them become enriched financially in any way that has no relation to your scope of practice.

Selling products, nutritional supplements, drinks, potions and programs should be carefully considered. Let me explain why.

Number One: As previously noted you do have undue influence over them- we want to believe everyone's an adult and can make their own decisions, but the facts most likely are,you are in a therapeutic type relationship where your student is seeking to please you – do things that you approve of. It may be uncomfortable, but it is like a parent-child relationship- sounds creepy and you may not want to believe it's true- but it is ! and also it is a somewhat necessary arrangement in order for you to be their teacher- it's the way it works, For the most part you can't change this- but your sacred obligation as a professional is to take great care with that power.

Number Two: If you do decide to enter into a secondary relationship with them, *(and believe me having Dual relationships with students is tricky)* the secondary relationship being- supplier of a product ….

if that product doesn't quite work-out the way you touted....

if they don't really like X Y or Z as much as you love it…

You have forever put a ding in your professional relationship with them.

There is a broken level of trust-that no matter what, you will never get back. They doesn't even need to be a horrible physical consequence to the situation- just the perception of "it wasn't as great as my teacher said it would be" is enough for their trust in whatever you say or do as their teacher to be questioned… when the trust in your abilities is gone- the teaching is done.

So what if you really like a product and want to share? You could consider presenting it in the most gentle way-soft sell, not making any financial gain, and just sharing your experience of it… and if you really feel selling some multi-level marketing product for financial gain is what you want to do, you can do that -but please consider that, what I have presented here, are the cold hard facts of the matter.

You can either be the wonderful supplier of a product you really believe in or a trusted teacher - very rarely can you be both. You must decide who you really want to be- both paths are fine, but to be a professional teacher -never ignore your sacred obligation to your student.

What about a product that is your own creation… basically same thing goes, but things like your dvd or ebook or special Pilates mat bags you sew-up in your spare time, do not pose as much of a conflict- They like how you teach- they'll enjoy your dvd. So really consider all sides of this issue before making a product pitch to your students.

TRAINING FRIENDS and FAMILY:

We've all experienced difficulties with trying to train and work with family and friends and/or becoming friends or maybe more with clients. Sometimes these relationships work…but most times they do not. The important thing to learn is the "why", and then from there with complete awareness decide whether those are the kinds of relationships you choose to develop.

Every time we agree to train a client -we are entering into several relationships.

1.**The Business Relationship**- you provide a service, they provide compensation for your time and expertise,-this is a somewhat equal relationship.

2.**The Therapeutic Relationship**- in this relationship they trust you are the expert, your position is elevated over theirs and there fore you have a certain amount of influence or power over them. (this is a sacred responsibility-treat it respectfully) this is not an equal relationship…. something subconscious happens here- they begin to view you through the lens of past relationships where they were dependent on someone- a parent, teacher, spouse, no one does this on purpose but it does happen- and depending on the nature good, bad, functional, dysfunctional - you have just become a player.

If you know this ahead of time you will be so far ahead of the game. You never want to tell a client, well your reacting like this because this is how you reacted to your mother, father, husband etc. - That's not important... The important thing is to remember that some of your clients reactions have nothing to do with you - don't take it personally. (Unless,of course, it does have something to do with you! So be professional always!) So if we're doing good work and not taking everything personally, the best course of action is, to take that subconscious dependency, and lead them toward a path of healthy independence. One where they enjoy your guidance and input but trust themselves to plot the journey.

3. **The Personal Relationship**- So with the complicated nature of the client-teacher relationship if you now chose to add another twist-another type of relating to each other , another type of relationship.....beware and be careful.

When you become friends with your clients a few complex issues will arise. Friends are generally equals- that's the way it works best... remember a therapeutic relationship is not a relationship of equals -so can you maintain the therapeutic relationship in the studio or class?

Will the student allow you back into the authority position when training?- Surprisingly this is difficult for them and maybe you - without the therapeutic aspect you might as well just become workout buddies- you can't train them !

Additionally you can never be truly your worst self with them.... like you are with your family or friends. You can't throw tantrums, and whine about stuff and make outrageous claims like- "I'm losing my mind"- Without risking their loss of trust in you. *(very scary for your client you hang upside down in fuzzies!)*

You need to treat their trust in you with kit gloves, as the teacher it is your sacred responsibility.

Lastly, let's be honest why do we become friends with clients and students?

I know you want to say it's our mutual interest and love of Pilates -but deeper than that, the fact is the work we do can sometimes be lonely, leaving little time for outside interests and we have to go out of our way to find those unrelated-to-our-work social occasions.

So be honest if you make your clients your friends because you're lonely acknowledge it (that's not to say we don't really like our clients-we do!).

You must STOP yourself whenever you find yourself asking the client to attend to your needs. They can talk and talk about their horrible relationships- but we should not …not ever…

The teacher does not look to the student for support- unless you don't care about damaging the relationship.

As for family and friends becoming clients the problem here is that they've already seen you whine and tantrum- they've been your equal for years and now you ask them to become less than equal - no wonder they are so difficult.

They will break all your rules, they will try to get away with things no regular student would - it's all a sub-conscious battle to maintain an equal standing with you.

The only way to train friends and family is to lay out the rules and do not deviate

- both parties need to agree… the training relationship and familial relationship are separate

- they exist totally apart- at home we don't discuss training and in our lesson we don't discuss home… we have set lesson times- no late shows- no staying late and hang out socializing

- otherwise the work will not get done and you have become an ineffectual teacher.

This is just a brief overview of the Client/friend problem. To recap: it is difficult and in many cases impossible but when attempting the dual relationship in a Pilates training setting some basic guidelines are:

1. Acknowledge there are concerns and difficulties that need to be consciously addressed

2. Set the rules and framework with clarity- times, fees, goals

3. Pilates session and social time are separate and never invade each others space

4. With the client who became the friend- be the strong together teacher they think you are-AT ALL TIMES, regardless!

5. Never ask for your needs to be met by the student- you need to cry on someone else's shoulder.

6. If your friends become clients -they must allow you to be the boss and follow your rules - or send them to someone else- you want them to get results- if you want to chat - go to lunch!

Again this is just dipping our toes into this
subject. Part of being a Professional is to
understand the nature of the business, therapeutic,
and ethical relationships we all encounter and how to
appropriately manage these. If you don't manage them-
they will manage you- and you will get burned and
burnt out.

MONEY BOUNDARIES:

 Seriously this is a scary and delicate topic for most of us. You probably started out in this field - not to make money… as if that's some disgusting horrible motivation! *(by the way, if you don't make money- you will need another job…)*

When I started pursuing my passion- teaching people movement- I'd often explain to people how I got the opportunity by being at a point in my life, where I didn't need to make money…as some sort of a justification.

Lesson: Don't feel guilty about making money doing what you're good at, what you love to do! Not being appropriately compensated in a financial way will burn you out !

When you work- you give your energy, and always that energy should be reciprocated… almost always that should take the form of - yes… money.

The money topic is sensitive mainly because we have distorted preconceptions and need to get comfortable with it's reality and purpose in our profession lives. Your misconceptions could be hurting your client relationships and business and impeding your ability to do good work.

A lot of the time movement teachers have very little business training. Those with a background always seem to thrive in this area. But have no fear- I will take you through some basic rules- which if you apply them- will take most of the stress out of the money issue.

Money does evoke strong feelings, both for you and your client. Therefore clear boundaries on your part, will not only help you- but will help them as well. Clients need strong clear boundaries about your policies and relationship- this allows the therapeutic/healing/growing relationship to exist and grow.

When your policies are wishy-washy, when you are not clear, you create an unsafe space for the client. They don't know what to expect. How can they trust you in any other way?

So here are some basic stumbling blocks and solutions.

1. My reward is the progress and healing I give to others….

If you feel this way, let me enlighten you to a reality. It has been shown that people will progress and heal more readily in a situation where they have had to give something to get something… it gives the thing they receive value. Even ancient healers and shaman asked for some sort of sacrifice or remuneration. So every time you discount or give away your services- you are making them less effective… it may be in the clients mind or subconscious, but isn't that *most* where it counts.

2. What to charge?

If you charge too little .. your clients will think your work may not be as good as others in your field, and your colleagues will be upset with your under-cutting- you damage the brand. If you charge too much-your clients make think you must be the best or maybe you're a price gouger- especially when they find out their friend goes to your colleague who is less pricey. Your colleagues will probably think you're a little full of yourself- especially if you're fairly new … so go with the flow BE COMFORTABLE AND CONFIDENT with your fees. (Unless you ARE %&*#$$ Awesome- then go for it!)

3. BE CONFIDENT

You must be comfortable with your fees and money policies. If you feel you must apologize, you need to truly examine- why? You must be straight-forward, sure and unapologetic. Your tone makes all the difference.

4. Have a Written Policy

This should include your fees and written policy for late arrivals, no shows and cancellations. You should go over this and have the client sign it - one for you -one for them.

5. Cancellations:

If your policy is to charge for late cancels (generally less than 24 hrs in advance) they cannot be shocked and you should not be apologetic... you're not selling Pilates, exercise or movement- you sell your time ! Listen again-**you sell your TIME...** if someone takes a time slot - you will not be selling that slot to anyone else. And even though you turned away someone 2 days prior -when they cancel 2 hours before- they just cost you money! Imagine their response if they showed up for a lesson and you booked someone else in their time slot- and expected them to still pay-took their money!? That would never work! Remember you are selling time slots and spaces - have a policy -stick to it...your clients will feel safer and know you are a professional who expects to be valued for your time- if they don't... you need to fire them!

6. ANY Changes to fees and policies need to be addressed with advance notice

If you will be changing your fees or policies - and I advise -do this with forethought and not too frequently … let your clients know with advance notice and again be confident and unapologetic…. it's business…. changing too frequently or with no notice makes your clients feel unsafe - you will lose clients this way… create a safe space.

7. Special Deals

Offering special deals all the time is a red flag to the consumer that somethings not right…. Also offering special deals to certain clients, (maybe you feel they can't afford you and you want to help) can be detrimental.

Yes it can be a bad thing… you are creating a dual relationship- not only are you their Pilates teacher- you are also their financial adviser now? Really, are you ready and willing for that responsibility? And when they come in and tell you about the vacation they planned for next month or some other expense they felt mattered more than their health… how will you feel? Resentful? Probably.

Can you really give a good lesson to someone who you are resenting?…hmmmm -pretty difficult. Resist giving the deal… (*to senior centers, schools, veterans -these may be exceptions) Resist giving the deal to generally able-bodied adults. You are creating a situation where you are enabling behaviors that say… I need special help, I can't function in the real world and follow the rules everyone else does… and you are not doing them any favors.

We all must desire and be willing to give something or give something up to receive health… otherwise it is a cheap commodity -and you and I know that's not true.

Ultimately receiving your compensation for the work you do- is the kindest and one of the most powerful exchanges you make with your client. You are making a contract that says -I will be a professional, I will use my knowledge to help you, as a professional -you can trust me to be discreet and ethical. In order to be an effective and powerful movement and wellness teacher- you must be a professional and all which that entails.

KEEPING CONFIDENCE:

It should go without saying but let's say it anyway...never talk about your students to other students, friends, families or teachers.

Now with all the "stuff" they share with you- you may feel over-whelmed. This can be stressful. They could be breaking your rules -this could be stressful. When your work stresses you out - you get burnt out! So what to do?

Create a confidential mentor relationship. This is a person that you can go to and vent! Blow off steam! Ask for advice and feedback. This person must be bound by confidentiality as well. This is your release valve. When we deal with others, we deal with their emotions and it will impact our own emotions.

You must set up this relationship.-on purpose. Discuss with the mentor, what you need and be sure that you feel they maintain a "safe space" for you.

When YOU create the "safe space" create the rules and boundaries - you will be more productive and less stressed out by your work. The "safe space"is healthy for you and the client.

CHECKPOINTS:

Define your policies in writing on these key issues:

Selling products

Fees

Fee Due Dates

Refunds

Cancellations

What constitutes a late cancellation?

Late Shows

No Shows

What do you promise to deliver for the fee?

Define your policy on confidentiality.

What happens if you need to late cancel?

Who will be your mentor, your release valve?

Having empathy for your student and their needs is important, but don't enable dependent behavior. You are here to help them become healthy- healthy IS independent self-empowerment.

We must be responsive to genuine concerns regarding movement and health.

We must realize that students come with emotional baggage that can impact their perceived physical limitations and progress - we are sensitive to that - but not over-whelmed.

We must be ready to refer students with emotional needs and issues beyond our professional scope to the appropriate professionals. Or refer students who's emotional baggage impairs our own ability to fully professionally deal with them to other teachers more suited to their situation.

SCIENCE OF THE ENERGETIC BODY

Your can be impacted by your work, physically,
mentally, emotionally and energetically.
You have a definable and real energetic body. The
human body has an electromagnetic energy field which
is measurable scientifically.

The human body is made of atoms and atoms are made up
of protons, neutrons and electrons.
Protons have a positive charge, neutrons have a
neutral charge, and electrons have a negative charge.

Atoms become either positively or negatively charged
when these charges are out of balance. When there is
a switch between one type of charge to the other,
this allows electrons to flow from one atom to
another. This flow of electrons, or a negative
charge, is what we call electricity.

At Yale, H.S. Burr's , in the 1930s produced a hard
data to support the hypothesis of the bio-electric
field as having unexplained qualities and acting as a
causal agent in development, healing, mood and
health.

Burr set up a series of experiments, later repeated
by other researchers, which demonstrated some
properties of these EM fields which he called Life-
fields (L-fields).

His experiments demonstrated that changes in the
electrical potential of the L-field were associated
with changes in the health of the organism.

Scientist and researcher Robert O Becker documented that human bodies generally carry a positive charge in the brain and spinal cord and a negative charge in the limbs.(Body Electric)

Negativity is the natural resting state of your cells, because there is an imbalance between potassium and sodium ions inside and outside the cell, and this imbalance sets the stage for your electrical capacity.

A Negative charge has more electrons. When something with a more electrons encounters something with less electrons.... the thing with less- takes, steals electrons from the thing with more. Nature is always seeking an equilibrium.

One of the most obvious evidences of our energetic body is simply the brain and nervous system. A vast complex of electrical impulses, far more complex that of any machine made by man. We are just now beginning to understand the complexity of the wiring- one of the current studies being the Human Brain Mapping Project -The Organization for Human Brain Mapping (OHBM) is the primary international organization dedicated to using neuro-imaging to discover the organization of the human brain.

So realizing that our body has an energetic aspect, which helps regulate our well-being **AND** that this energetic aspect reacts inside, outside and around our bodies - like any other energetic field in our physical world- it can be of no surprise that your energetic field, my energetic field and that of our clients are interacting on the atomic level with each other at the very least when we come in close proximity to each other.

After much study, research and personal experience, it is this author's opinion that we do affect our clients -energetically and that they in turn can affect us.

We've all had that friend, family member or client that left us drained and exhausted after spending some time with them. We've felt like they sucked the life out of us. News flash! They did! They literally stole your electrons.

Chances are they were down, depressed, negative or in ill-health. Of course you started out feeling pretty good, positive upbeat, but soon you could feel your energy being drained away, your mood changing and you had no idea, why?

After a while you may look for ways to avoid these people- it's a survival mechanism. Being around these energy vampires on a regular basis without knowing how to guard your energy is detrimental to your own health.

Working with clients there will generally always be somewhat of an energy transfer. You need to know how to manage that , how to guard your energy and how to restore your energy.

Hopefully -you are not the one with the energy deficit! If you are, you should not be working with clients. You know when you are depleted, burnt out- you can not do your best work, you can not even do good work. Not only does the client get short-changed. You might also be a drain on their energy!

If you are working at a deficit- it is imperative for you to restore your balance. If you feel like you need a good long vacation... this is a red flag. Maybe you can't take a vacation right now. You can still re-balance yourself.

When working with clients, make certain you have created the the "safe space" rules and expectations all defined and adhered to.

Next when meeting with any client be fully mentally present, assess their energy and attitude, so you can make wise decisions on your level of interaction.

Keep your perspective, listen carefully and closely- but keep a good perspective. Being compassionate and open is important but if you find yourself over-identifying with their issues- physical or otherwise - it's time to take a step back.

One of the major places you give off electrons are your hands, so by bringing your hands together or crossing your arms, while you interact is a good way to begin a session.

Of course - you will not hold your hands and arms like this for the entire session, but begin like this.

Please note if you opt to cross the arms keep them at a low level on your body- not across the chest which appears closed off and makes you appear too guarded. This position is also a good restorative and can be practiced throughout your day.

Be aware - if someone's bad mood, serious issue or general negativity starts to affect you make a mental note, keep your own outlook positive, maintain a balancing posture- keep your physical cues and touch to an absolute minimum.

Make it a point to do restorative energy work on yourself as quickly after the session as possible.

When we tactility cue, when we touch to direct, we relay directional information and there will be an exchange of electrons. Done with a positive intention this can deliver a positive and perhaps profound response. If we are keeping our bodies and minds healthy and balanced - there are electrons to spare -so we give them some of ours, they feel better and if you are aware of restoring yourself- you won't fear- because t**he universe is full of energy!** *(by the way- the majority of it- IS FREE)*

There are times when a clients poor energy management make them a liability to your good health- you might need to fire them.

Think of it like this, if you worked in a space full of asbestos or other cancer causing chemicals – would you stay?

If you find yourself unable to maintain and restore balance around a particular client... you must let them go .

Each time you are drained by them, you get a little more depleted physically and mentally and pretty soon you might be of no help what-so-ever to anyone. Start tuning into your body, trusting your gut, trusting your instinct. Your nervous system (which is electrical !) is sending messages to your brain every second. It's your job to listen up!

Our senses know when we are in danger or creating unhealthy situations for ourselves. Have you stopped listening?

The most compassionate caring thing you can do for your clients is to keep yourself healthy physically, mentally, emotionally and energetically. In that way you can provide them with superior instruction from a balanced and aware perspective.

METHODS FOR RESTORATION:

Completing your own circuit:
Cross the arms low over the body, or better clasp the hands together palms touching, placing the hands together prayer position is a good way to restore energy...you don't need to be praying to gain benefit (if you want to -go ahead) either way there is great benefit- a minimum of 5 minutes . (you can do this exercise 1, 2, 3 or several times per day)

Toes in the Grass!
Go outdoors, barefoot stand on the ground, grass , beach, dirt, whatever just not pavement...stand on the earth - no shoes - minimum of 5 minutes. The earth resonates at about 7.8hz, the human being between 7hz and 8hz. The human body is only capable of responding beneficially and healthfully to a small slice of the electromagnetic frequency spectrum. Working indoors, with lots of electronic devices, lights, driving a car you are exposed to energy fields much higher than our bodies are designed for. So go outside and re-balance your energy.

Take a Salt water bath or go jump in the ocean if you can! :
Since the time of Hippocrates this has been prescribed for all kinds of ailments of body and mind. Salt bathing works partly because natural mineral salts restore mineral balance through the skin. It is well known that the skin can absorb medicines and chemicals. Natural salt contains many minerals, including magnesium, which helps the nervous system, balancing your electrical energy. It can relieve stress, and can relieve water retention. Bromides in the salt heal and relax your muscles.

Create rituals that restore your energy.
There is nothing wrong with rituals. Humans need ritual.

In some cultures rituals and practices like feng-shui or ritual clearings that are performed in a space to balance the energy and restore positivity. Practices like smudging and using crystals may be meaningful to you and as such should be employed .

When your intention is to create balance and good health in your life , the path you take to get there is far less important than actually getting out your walking shoes and taking that walk.

Your way- is the right way for you. You can explore these various practices and if they help set your frame of mind on the positive -then these are the correct tools for your journey. Create meaningful rituals for yourself. Honor the energetic you.

Part Two

Grow your business with 6 steps to SASS !

What is SASS?
SASS is Steps Above Service System.

Are you delivering service which is "Steps Above"
your competition?

If you consistently do deliver superior service, if
you have a plan of action and work that plan every
workday.
You will be successful.

BEARS REPEATING- Work that plan **EVERY** day!

To deliver superior service you must be able to
first, design and implement workout strategies that
work! If you fail at this first step- all the rest of
your efforts will be for naught.

So make *absolutely sure* you have received the best
training yourself and continue to hone your skills on
a regular basis.

The Step Above Service plan starts the moment the client meets you.

Initial Contact !

There are 2 parts to the intake:

The History and Goal-setting!

A full and complete health and lifestyle history should be taken at the initial meeting. You must understand the clients starting point, any contraindications or lifestyle issues that will affect your program design.

MOST IMPORTANTLY:

Goals of the client should be clearly understood, let them tell you everything, everything!
Then ASK them what results they expect from training with you?

Only then do you understand what they want.
Only then, can you decide if you can deliver what they expect..

Design a workout program with pre-scheduled re-assessment appointments at regular intervals. It seems like common sense and maybe you are re-assessing and course correcting at each appointment but this is **even more** for the client's benefit than for yours.

If you are new to training, the process of formally re-assessing gives you direction. Are you heading towards your goals, their goals, or are you treading water?

Even if you are certain you are making progress, your client needs clear data to see that happening too.

People pay you to progress. If you provide tangible proof of their progress it is motivating and encourages adherence and commitment.

Clear record keeping of lesson plans, benchmarks and progress not only makes your job easier it helps maintain the "safe space" … these are the parameters, these are the boundaries.

Providing a regular written report card of a client's progress, is a tangible reminder for them, that keeping appointments and doing their homework - works!

Speaking of homework, every student should receive
homework, unless you are seeing them 3 to 4 times a
week.

Homework, ideally is written down .

Will they do the homework? If they are committed to
their own health- yes!
If not.....keep giving homework and asking if they've
done it.

If they see you less than 3 times per week, they NEED
homework to make sufficient progress. It is important
for you to have this discussion with them, otherwise
they may believe seeing you for 60 minutes a week
will give them a whole new physique......unlikely!

The foundation of your service should be setting and
meeting the client's goals, with a personalized
effective workout and homework with regular progress
reports .

This is the foundation. To provide SASS and rise
above the rest you need to go above and beyond this!
To be a step above...go to the the step above, aim
higher, commit to a level above, with each
client....every-time.

Deliver more than expected !

Provide the little extras- the nicety's that tell
your client that they are in good and caring hands.

Provide additional education and resources, it says
to your client that you are dedicated to empowering
them to improve their health.

The little extras that can mean a whole lot!

Some ideas to show your client you appreciate them and their business.

1.A Thank You card sent when they initially sign-up OR at anytime of the year to let them know you are grateful for their patronage. This should always be sent in the regular mail. An email though pleasant doesn't convey this message in the same meaningful way.

2.Client appreciation week. A week where each client gets a small gift and a thank you card, maybe the studio provides special refreshments and visibly announces through posters and banners how much you appreciate your clients.

3.Birthday cards!

4.Free bottled water? The cost is nominal and providing this, when other gyms and studios charge $2 and $3 dollars a bottle can seem like a luxury.

5.Our studio also puts out free granola bars, raisins and other snacks.

6.Congratulate and celebrate reaching goals! A card, a note, a balloon or balloon bouquet . Reinforcing , how good it feels to be successful- breeds more drive and therefore more success- help create an upward lift, where once there was a downward spiral.

7.Create an atmosphere that is welcoming, Be happy to
see your client.

8.Do all the nice things and still stick to your guns
when it comes to policy.
 It says-"I really care about you and your health and
the best way for me to provide you with the success
you want and deserve is by creating the "safe space."

9.Provide personalized written homework.

10.If they see other health professionals or see
other trainers when they travel provide documentation
of their current program and assessments.

Educate and Inform

Often the client enlists the help of others- in the
form of trainers, therapists and doctors, but they
forget the most important member of their wellness
team is them.

Guide them to see - they need to get on their own
team... guide them to take charge of that team and
take their rightful place as team captain.

Providing education about Pilates, fitness and exercise in the form of regularly distributed handouts is a great way to empower the client to take ownership in their success.

If you are fairly adept at writing, send out a monthly e-newsletter or write a blog.

Direct clients to websites with content you approve, by emailing links or providing a monthly list in the studio.

Start out by planning 3 months of education for your clients, each month exploring one unique topic.

*Provided on the next few pages are 3 handouts which you may copy and re-distribute, to get you started. Don't be afraid- design your own informative handouts or provide copies of important health-related articles you find online or in print. *Remember to get appropriate permission from the author to duplicate and give credit to the writer.*

What Are the Principles of Pilates? And how do they help me?

There are several key principles of Pilates. Major schools, organizations and leaders across the globe agree on most.

The first principle is **Breath** ! Joseph Pilates said, "breath is the first act of life and the last". True, and profound. It is a vitally important aspect of doing Pilates which helps move and coordinate the exercises and helps the student mentally direct their energy to the task at hand. So when your teacher gives cues for breathing, listen and try to incorporate those directions into your movement.

The next principle is **Concentration**. Your mind should be fully engaged in the moment. Do not let your attention wander to other details of your day, or distractions around you. This is a tough practice ! Pilates long ago, before it was the fashion and catch-phrase, knew what Mind-Body meant. Development of a fit body is inter-twined with development of a sound mind. Learn to be the master of your mind through the use of Pilates techniques.

A third principle is **Control**. Are you in "control" of your body, of your movements. Do you walk, sit and stand with surety and purpose? Or are you slouchy through life as your body slowly disintegrates and falls apart. To feel healthy and vigorous – you need to have control.

Number four: muscular development **Balance**. A body uniformly (as possible) developed has less stress at the joints, it feels better and maybe more importantly to you -it looks better. When you improve your posture through even body conditioning you look younger and taller !

The last principle we will explore is **Whole Body Movement**. There is no exercise in Pilates in which your entire body doesn't play a role. Every exercise starts from a strong powerhouse, center and radiates outward... let your whole body and mind participate in the exercise... and then move , flow and one more thing.....do it joyfully. Even when it's hard, frame of mind matters.

So remember:
Breathe, Concentration , Control , Muscle Balance ,Whole Body Movement

As Joseph Pilates said, "Physical fitness is the first requisite of happiness. Our interpretation of physical fitness is the attainment and maintenance of a uniformly developed body with a sound mind fully capable of naturally, easily, and satisfactorily performing our many and varied daily tasks with spontaneous zest and pleasure."

written by: Laurette Ryan

Distributed by:

Pre-Pilates Exercises to Improve your Performance !

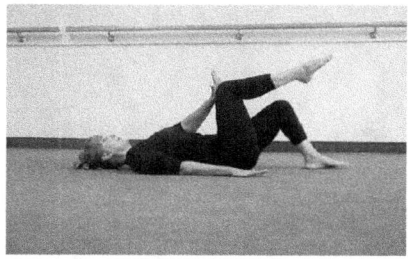

ALTERNATE KNEE PRESS-
Lie on your back,

Bring one knee up to a table top position towards the
chest and press the opposite palm against it -resisting
and tightening the abs at the same time. Pulling the abdominals inward.
Do not let the belly bulge!

Repeat on the other side and hold each time for 10 seconds.
4 to 10X each side.

This exercise contracts the abdominal in an isometric manner.
It is safe for most every fitness level and very effective.

CHAIR LEG PRESS AND LOWER-
Lie on your back,
Legs in a tabletop position both up, keeping the pelvis and spine stable .
(not moving)

Extend one leg out and gently lower it 2 to 4 inches
Still maintaining a stable hip (pelvis) and back (spine) . Keep the belly flat
– no bulging!

Repeat on the other side-
4-10 X each side.

*This is a more challenging exercise . When you are able to do this with
ease , you may want to progress to extending both legs simultaneously.
Attention discomfort in the spine is indication to ease back or stop. Listen
to your body. You ARE the boss of it!

Written by: Laurette Ryan

Distributed by:

Pilates Builds Fascial Fitness

The buzz word in fitness lately is fascia! What you need to know is fascia is just about everywhere- throughout you're whole body. You my friend are a fascial bubble!

Without going into the long biology of it all. Suffice to say you're body is constantly building, rebuilding, breaking down, remolding and remodeling you -all the time. Honestly, it does it a bit slower as we age , but if you can re-build, remodel yourself into the the best body possible- why wouldn't you? Look better, have less pain and ease of everyday activities – it's a great goal.

Pilates done regularly and with care and attention will improve your fascial fitness by it's very nature.

Why? Well the parameters of Pilates training are the parameters a fitness and exercise program need to incorporate to achieve this very powerful aspect of health.

1.Whole Body Movements- Pilates IS whole body movement –
   every exercise should incorporate your whole body.

2.Fascia is nerve Rich – Talk to the Sensory Organ----Fascia!
   The mind-body concentration of Pilates helps a person tune into the deep movements of the tissues -not just make a bulging bicep in the gym mirror.

3.Proximal Initiation-
   In Pilates one should always begin by move from the center.

4.Move in Opposition to Prepare.
   There is direction to – push down to go up and reach up to go down throughout Pilates -it is natural and reinforced in the practice.

5.Move with Elasticity
   Movements flow in Pilates , there is no herky-jerky ,heavy impact.

6.Variation in Movement Patterns-
   Working from the center, using different levers (arms & legs) and body positions . Using natural , sensible and variable movements.

7.Varying Load and Tempo-
   Each exercise has a rhythm and variety in Springs, Apparatus ,Props and cuing is essential to achieve the goal.

Joseph Pilates said, **"Contrology is not a system of haphazard exercises designed to produce only bulging muscles. ... Nor does Contrology err either by over-developing a few muscles at the expense of all others with resulting loss of grace and suppleness, or a sacrifice of the heart or lungs. Rather, it was conceived to limber and stretch muscles and ligaments so that your body will be as supple as that of a cat and not muscular like that of the body of a brewery-truck horse, or the muscle-bound body of the professional weight lifter you so much admire at the circus."**

Written by: Laurette Ryan

Distributed by:

Lastly you should develop a network of trusted professionals. These are people you feel confident in referring to. They might include massage therapists, physical therapists, general practitioners, chiropractors, nutritionists and counselors.

So to summarize your SASS (Step Above Service System)

1. Design and Personalize the workout plan.

2. Provide Homework

3. Written Progress Reports

4. Special nicety's

5. Extra Education and resources

6. Be Professional
    and all which that entails 100% of the time!

Thank You, I hope that these ideas help you create a stress-free rewarding business.

If you would like pdf copies of the handouts please feel free to email me at Laurette@balancepointstudios.com .

Happy to be of assistance!

Wishing you peace and prosperity!

Laurette Ryan

www.ingramcontent.com/pod-product-compliance
Lightning Source LLC
Chambersburg PA
CBHW081119290526
45795CB00006B/2177